There Is
No Magic Pill

The Healthy Way To Lose Weight, And Keep It Off For Good

R. SUE OLESON

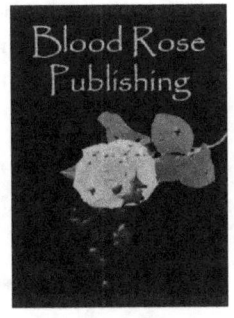

Blood Rose Publishing

FIRST EDITION
ISBN: 150787667X
ISBN-13: 978-1507876671

A WORD OF CAUTION

This book is intended to be used as a guideline for starting your path to a healthier way of eating and losing weight. It was inspired by our own personal journey to getting fit, losing weight, and living a healthier lifestyle.
It was written to give others an idea of how food works in our bodies, and how the choices we make can affect our overall health and wellness. It is not intended to serve as a substitute for any instruction or advice given to any reader by their physician.
As always, consult your physician for any health issues you may have, and the author strongly recommends that you follow any instruction or recommendation of your physician, over any advice or information you may receive from this book.

CONTENTS

FORWARD

Let me start by saying that I am, by no means, any kind of expert. I am not a nutritionist; I am not a fitness expert, or a personal trainer. I am a regular person, just like you. I am a Registered Nurse, and I used what knowledge I have learned from that profession – about health, diet, and exercise – along with research and a lot of willpower, to get where I wanted to be in my own personal journey. In less than a year, my husband and I together lost almost 100 pounds; almost two years later, we have kept that weight off, and we are getting better every day. We have no intentions of going back to the way things were. So many people have asked us, *"How did you do it?"* And when we would tell them, they would say, *"No, really. What are you taking?"* Our honest and simple answer to these people was, and still is, *"There is no magic pill."* My husband then suggested since I am already a published author, I should write down what worked so well for us; and so the idea for this book was born.

The next thing that I want to say is this: STOP RIGHT HERE if you are not completely committed to making a 'lifestyle change'. This is not a 'diet'. It takes commitment and dedication and will-power. It is a

CHANGE, and most people do not like change. You WILL see results, but only if you are *honest* with yourself and with the plan I am going to share with you; and if you are *committed* to making the change. In the beginning, it is a lot of *work* – not *hard* work, but it is work. It *will* make a difference – but *not* without *you*. You are the deciding factor. Your willingness to stick to the plan will be your success or your failure. If you are *not* at your wit's end – if you are *not* dedicated to making the necessary changes – you *will* fail. And until you are ready for such a commitment, you might as well not read any further. Should you choose to continue reading, even if you are not ready at this point, I can only refer to the old adage: *"You can lead a horse to water, but you can't make him drink."*

For those of you that are still with me: let me finish this opening statement by saying that you may see, in this book, references to products and brands. I am not, by any means, endorsing or favoring any particular brand or product over another; and there is no intent, on my part, to encourage or entice any reader to buy any certain product or brand that may be mentioned, over another, or even at all. I am merely giving reference to what I have tried, and what I have found worked best for me. As consumers, each one of you is highly encouraged to do your own research, to find what works for *you*; something you know you will enjoy and *stick with*.

That being said, I wish you the best of luck in your journey to a healthier, more fit, and hopefully, a happier 'you'.

HOW IT STARTED

I have never been what you would consider to be a 'large' person, or what most would call 'fat'. But like most women, I have a long-standing love / hate relationship with my body. My weight, over the years, as well as my body shape, has fluctuated. But until the most recent few years, my highest body weights have been during pregnancies.

Likewise, my husband – who was 220 pounds when I met him – while large, would not be considered 'fat', given his stature of six-foot-three. As it turns out, one of the things we had in common, when we met, was a love of good food. I cooked 'comfort food' at home, and nights out always included dinner at a steak house – a big, juicy steak along with all the trimmings: salad slathered in dressing, loaded baked potato, and a nice, fluffy yeast roll bathed in melted butter.

In the early years of our relationship, I took a management-level job which required me to work long hours; even when I was scheduled off, I was still on-call, and my phone rang quite frequently. In fact, there were not many times that we could find ourselves making it all the way through a meal without me getting a phone call.

The position was, to say the least, very high stress. Because of my hectic schedule, it became easier and easier for us to just eat out all of the time.

When I decided to leave that position after almost a decade, what I found in my job search were more employers wanting to hire me for the same level position. They valued my experience as a manager, and were hesitant to hire me into a lower-level position. To that end, I decided to go in a different direction in my career. This meant starting at the bottom of the totem pole – which translated in the nursing world, means working the night shift.

Working all night, while my family was sleeping, and sleeping during the day while they went to work / school, now meant that our social time had to be more scheduled and structured. I found that one of the most enjoyable times to spend with my family meant eating food. Getting off work at seven a.m., as they were waking for the day, meant I could get home and cook some waffles and sausage, or pick up some donuts or other fast-food breakfast. Everyone's favorite seemed to be breakfast burritos. A local convenience store has a deli of sorts, where you can get a breakfast burrito loaded so full of meat, eggs, cheese, and potatoes, the tortilla will not even stay wrapped around it!

Eating like this each morning, and then falling into bed for an eight- to ten-hour stretch, did not help matters with my weight. Not to mention that after sleeping all day, I would get up, shower, and dress for work, just in time for us to go out to eat, before I had to report for duty. And anyone that has ever worked a night shift will tell you that one of the things you do, to stay alert and awake all night, is snack.

The changes were barely noticeable at first – at least I

thought. I knew some of my clothes felt a little tighter. But my husband has always been wonderful about telling me how beautiful and sexy I look, and at first I didn't even mind a few extra pounds. I could easily throw on scrubs, or jeans and a T-shirt, and be comfortable, and – or so I thought – hide the extra pounds I had packed on. The realization that this was not the case hit me during a series of events.

My birthday falls in December. Hubby said we could do anything I wanted for my birthday. A local theater group was presenting "The Nutcracker Suite." I had never been to the ballet, and didn't really think he would agree. But he did. So I bought tickets for the show, and made reservations at an upscale restaurant we had never tried before. I was so excited about my upcoming date night for my birthday. And then I went shopping.

I made three different shopping trips in as many weeks, trying – at first – to find something *special* to wear. Later, after being reduced to many tears, I changed my quest to a goal of finding *anything* that looked half-way decent on my much-larger body. I found an outfit, but I was not completely satisfied with it. The blouse didn't lay right over my increased chest size. My heels hurt my feet, and even made my toes go numb! But I suffered through my special night – which of course, included a large meal with wine and dessert – with a smile on my face.

Later that same month, we attended my husband's company Christmas dinner, after which, someone posted pictures of us on Facebook. *Oh, my goodness! Look at how fat my face looks! My face!* That was what I saw, even though there were many comments from family and friends, saying how beautiful I looked. Of course, we are all our own worst critics, right? I was only seeing what I wanted to see. There was no way I was as large as those pictures made it seem that I was. And everyone knows that the camera adds a few pounds! Fast-forward to February, which brought a cousin's wedding. This meant another tortured shopping spree, and another event to which I wore, what I considered to be, less-than-desirable clothing choices. But by this time, I had begun to feel 'okay' with the extra pounds I was carrying; until, again – I saw the pictures. These were even more horrifying to me than those from Christmas.

And now I had to face the facts. I was now heavier than I had ever been in my life (without the benefit of being with child). Yes – I had gotten *fat – overweight – obese.* For someone my stature of five-foot-four, in medical terms, I *would* be considered obese.

I sat down to think about the past few years of my life. I thought about all the meals I had skipped because I was 'too busy' to stop and eat; only to have a large, heavy meal before watching an hour or two of TV, and then going straight to bed. I thought about how inactive and tired I had become. But I didn't have extra energy to do anything, other than work and go home. And I decided it was time to make a change. I didn't know how it was going to work, but by this time, I was bound and determined to try.

THE DECISION TO CHANGE

So how did I decide what to do? The most logical course of action, I concluded, was to look at what I had tried in the past – things I knew for sure would *not* work. I knew I needed to go a different route than anything I had ever tried before.

As I stated before, my weight has fluctuated over the years – because of having three children, as well as other significant life events. I knew fad diets did not work. I knew fasting did not work. I knew so-called 'diet pills' did not work. At one point in my life, I was even an 'exercise junky' – going to the gym religiously, *seven* days a week – and still did not see what I consider *significant* results.

When I really started to think about it, I knew I needed to start 'practicing what I preach'. As a nurse, how many times had I explained to a patient how to follow a heart-healthy diet? Or a diabetic diet? Or *any* special diet, for that matter? What did I already know about nutrition, which I hadn't bothered to practice in my own life? I also thought about my husband's eating habits as well. How was I going to approach him with this? Our schedules were so different at this time; I wasn't sure if he would stick to any sort of plan, when I wasn't around to carry it out for him. The more I thought about my situation, the more questions ran through my mind. Once I realized that all my questions were just excuses in disguise, I knew it was time to get started.

I can't even remember now what that last meal was that I prepared – but I made a great home-cooked dinner for 'the talk'. When we sat down at the table to eat – and my husband extolled of my fabulous cooking skills, as he heaped up his plate – I told him.

"Honey, I'm glad you like it, because this is the last time I think I'll ever cook this way for you."

When he asked what I meant, I told him of my decision. I explained how tired I felt, and how I was tired of always feeling tired. I felt tired when I went to bed; and yet, no matter how long I slept, I felt just as tired, if not more, when I woke up. And, I was tired of the way my clothes fit, and not feeling attractive – no matter *how many times* he told me how sexy and beautiful he thought I was – because I wasn't happy with *myself*.

I told him I wanted to eat better – to eat *healthier* – and that I intended to do it, no matter what. I explained that he would either have to be with me, or he would be on his own to fend for himself at mealtime. I might have to do this alone, but I had every intention of *doing it*.

When I finished, he sat there quietly for a moment. Then he looked at me and said "okay." He then admitted to me that he had been thinking the very same way about himself, but he just didn't know how to go about the change. He said if I planned it, he would go along with it, and he would leave our future health and nutrition in what he called my capable hands. He trusted my knowledge, and said he was more than willing to give it a try.

It has now been almost two years since we started this journey of making this lifestyle change, and we have lost a combined total of 94 pounds and 36 inches. These numbers would be somewhat larger, but while I opted for an exercise program that focused on toning and strengthening, my husband decided to take a more 'body-building' approach to his exercise regimen, which by its very nature, requires *adding* muscle weight and size. But I don't want to get ahead of you at this point – the option to exercise will be discussed later. For now, let's get back to the issue at hand – which is nutrition.

I could not decide for my husband, no more than I can make this decision for you. I could not make him join me on this journey. I could only extend the invitation, just as I am now doing with you, by way of sharing this information.

I've told you my reasons for going down this path. Now you must make that same decision. What are your reasons for wanting to lose weight? Is it for your looks and self-esteem? For the way you feel and for general health? And how badly do you want it? Are you willing to commit to making a change – for the better? You are the 'horse' in this story – and only *you* can decide at this point if you want to take that drink. In the end, only you can say whether or not you are thirsty enough.

START SMALL, PLAN BIG!

So much emphasis today, especially in the restaurant and fast-food industry, is placed on 'more'. Bigger portions of food, served on bigger plates; bigger cups for your drink, and "how much value can you get for mere dollars?"

What so many people fail to realize, is while they are getting 'more' for their money at this point in time, what does it cost them in the long run? How many of you stop to think – every time you eat a French fry – what the cost of cardiac care is? The cost of cholesterol medication? The cost of blood pressure medication? The cost of insulin and diabetic supplies? Not to mention the cost of each visit to the doctor's office, the specialist(s) you may be referred to for treatment of whatever ails you, and the cost of all the tests they will run – blood tests, stress tests, EKG's, and the like.

We are a nation that has been killing ourselves with food – too much of the *wrong* kinds of food, in ever-growing mega portions, along with a sedentary lifestyle. When you place the emphasis on eating the right kinds of foods, prepared the right way, and served in the right-sized portions, you will be *amazed* at the differences you will notice in your body in just mere days!

You will feel less sluggish. Your energy levels will go up. Your thought processes become clearer. Your memory will improve. You will rest better, because you will *sleep* better. And you will start to see the pounds slowly come off.

Wait a minute. You caught that, didn't you? Yes, I said *slowly*. This is not a fad diet, remember? This is a lifestyle change. What you have to realize is that the weight you lose in this manner will be so much more likely to stay off over time. What you gained over the course of years will take longer than mere weeks to lose. Following a healthy eating plan will allow you to lose it, and keep it off. Fad diets and weight-loss products so often fail because of several reasons. First, the menus tend to be extreme, and they don't allow for any kind of 'cheating', so you become more tempted to stray, and eventually, abandon the diet altogether. Second, they most often cause loss of more 'water weight' than fat loss; this weight loss isn't sustainable over time. And finally, they don't teach you how to change your own eating habits, a valuable tool you need for both preparing meals at home, and to make better choices when dining out. These fad diets and products virtually set you up for an inevitable failure. What is worse, when you start to gain back the weight, most people have a tendency to gain back *more* than where they first started. The rebounding, yo-yo effect of this type of weight loss can wreak as much havoc on your health as being overweight to begin with.

So how do you get started? First, you need to get rid of every negative thought about what it means to eat healthy – or rather, what most people have a tendency to think it means. Am I telling you that you can never eat a French fry, or a slice of pizza, ever again? Absolutely not! I'm going to tell you how to eat to lose weight, feel great, feel better about yourself, and *still* be able to enjoy these things! With very few exceptions, there is virtually *nothing* on a list of things you *must* give up.

The biggest part of making this change will be the advance-planning of meals, and maintaining portion control. You will also need to adjust your eating schedule to accommodate eating five to six meals per day. Later, I will explain why; but for now, I'll stick with helping you plan.

Start by cleaning out your kitchen – the refrigerator, the cabinets, and the pantry. Pick one or two items that you can use to 'reward' yourself, such as a bag of your favorite cookies or that box of microwave popcorn. But throw out the rest of the 'junk' – chips, pastries, cookies, crackers, processed food products such as ready-made dinners, canned soups or meals (ravioli, spaghetti-o's, mac-n-cheese, etc.). Get rid of it. Donate it to a food pantry. Give it to a neighbor or a co-worker in need. Or just trash it. Get it out of the house!

Next, make menus and a shopping list. Buy whole-grain breads and cereals, oatmeal, fresh fruits and vegetables, and fresh lean meats such as boneless, skinless chicken breast, ground turkey, fish fillets, and boneless pork steak or pork chops. Stock up on eggs, milk, and all-natural peanut butter.

Make sure you have a good set of measuring devices. You will need measuring cups for both liquid and dry measure, and measuring spoons. And you need to *use them*!

Separate bulk items into single-sized servings. Buy both snack-sized and sandwich-sized zip-lock bags, and small, serving-sized containers (both Glad® and Ziplock® make small, throw-away storage bowls that are perfect for this purpose). *Read* labels! If a serving of cereal is a half-cup, use a measuring cup and break the box of cereal down into half-cup servings (or use the measuring cup *every time* you eat that cereal). Do the same with baked chips or whole-grain crackers, such as Wheat Thins® or Triscuit® – if the box says six crackers is a serving, put six crackers in each container. I separated mine into snack-sized bags, and then put all the bags back into the box. When I wanted a snack, I knew I could just 'grab a bag' and that was a serving; I didn't have to worry about eating right out of the box and over-indulging.

Cook only enough for the number of people in your household who will be eating at each meal. A serving of meat – an *actual* serving of meat – is between four and six ounces. It is *not* the 12- or 16-ounce steak you get at the steakhouse! A good rule of thumb for meats is no bigger than the palm of your hand. And I'm not talking about a filet mignon here, which is around an inch thick, either – you don't get off that easy! *Four* to *six* ounces. If you need one to keep you on track, buy a small kitchen food scale. You can buy one at most major chain stores (WalMart, K-Mart, Target) for less than ten dollars. If you are cooking for two, prepare *two* chicken breasts, or *two* pork chops. No more – no seconds, no room for error.

The good news here? You are *not* going to starve! A serving of vegetables is two cups. That's right, I said *two* cups! And you may not even think that's a lot at this point, but wait until you try to eat two cups of steamed broccoli for the first time! What's that you say? You don't like broccoli? Tell me this, and the first thing I will ask you is, *"Have you ever tried it?"* If your answer is 'yes', the next thing I'm going to ask you is, *"How was it prepared?"*

No matter your answer, you have to go into this with an open mind. Before we started this journey, my husband would not eat anything 'green' if it was not lettuce or green beans – period. His idea of vegetables was corn and potatoes, cooked in any fashion. And the majority of things he said he 'didn't like' were things he had never actually tried. Variety is the key to a balanced healthy diet plan that you can stick with. And it's necessary for biology, but we will discuss those reasons in the next chapter.

Later, I will give you sample menus and meal plans, but one thing I'm *not* going to do is tell you *what* to eat. I'll leave that for you to decide on your own. I can only assume that you are an adult and capable of making your own decisions. And if you are here at this point already, I can also assume that you only need to be steered in the right direction. But if you are open-minded, and willing to expand your horizons, so to speak, you *will* have results – for the simple fact of that same biology.

WHY IT WORKS WITH THE BODY

Every person is different, and will see different results from following this plan, so I'm not going to tell you that you are 'guaranteed' to lose "x" amount of pounds in "x" amount of days. But one thing that is *not* different about all of us is biology. Sure, genetics can play some part; but just because your parents were 'fat' does not doom you to a lifetime of obesity.

Every part of the human body is made up of cells. Cells need energy, which comes in the form of food and hydration. When we eat food and drink liquids, our body reacts like a factory, breaking down everything we ingest, and sending the broken-down products where they are needed, or when not needed, they are stored for later. Different cells or body parts (organs) require different types of energy to function correctly, and most efficiently.

To put it in the simplest terms, think of your body as you would a car. You put gas in the car, and you expect it to run. But you can only go as far as that tank of gas will take you, and then you have to put more in. But suppose you are on a trip, and you have plenty of gas, but you get a flat tire. Air is different from gas. You have to put air in the tire to make the car run again, even though it already has gas, or you can greatly damage the car by driving it on a flat tire. The same goes with motor oil. You can have plenty of gas, and all four tires can be aired up, but if you lose motor oil, the engine will stop. Even though you have gas in the tank and air in the tires, that car isn't going anywhere!

When we deprive our bodies of the right kinds of energy for all the different types of cells to function, our bodies have to work harder and compensate. For the way most people eat these days, that compensation comes in the form of fat storage. And when I say fat storage, I'm not only referring to the fats you eat, but to *everything* you eat – fats, proteins and carbohydrates. The reason behind this is that everything you eat, that is *beyond* the amount required to sustain function, is stored by the body for later use *when necessary*. I use the term 'when necessary', because when you constantly overeat, and you give your body an over-abundance of fuel which it stores for later, and you do not *use* that fuel (in the form of some sort of exercise), you gain fat. If you were to literally starve yourself, your body would start to break down the stored fat to use as energy, because it is necessary to keep you alive. Once your fat stores are depleted, your body will start to break down muscle as an energy source. To maintain a constant weight, you must take in the same amount of calories that you expend in a day. To lose weight, you must take in fewer calories than required to maintain your current weight in a day, or you must expend more calories than you take in during the day. Although these may sound very similar, these are *two very different concepts* that we will explore when we talk about deciding to exercise.

Go back to my weight-gaining story. Remember how I said there were days that I just didn't have time to eat? How many of you have done that? I know I have skipped meals in the past because of 'being too busy', and I've also skipped meals in the past, hoping that not eating as much would help me shed a few pounds. But then, we go home toward the end of the day, and eat one huge meal. What you assume would happen – by eating only one meal per day – is to lose weight. However, the opposite effect is truer. Your body – your *metabolism* – will *adjust itself* to the energy you give it. By eating less, and depriving your body of needed energy, it is going to hold on to everything you put in when you finally feed it. In essence, I'm saying that to lose weight, you need to *eat more*! How great is that?

Now I'm not talking about a free-for-all here. This is not license to 'eat what you want, as much as you want'. I'm talking about eating the right kinds of foods throughout the day, in the proper portions, to sustain the highest efficiency of bodily function. When you start to follow the plan, your body – *and* your metabolism – will adjust itself accordingly; just as it did when you put it into starvation mode. When you give it food for energy, it wakes up and says, *"Hey, what is this?"* And it will use what it needs to function, and store whatever is left over. When you feed your body again in a few hours, it will say, *"Hey, I'm getting some more!"* Once your body decides that you are going to feed it on a regular basis, and give it the right kinds of foods it needs to function, it won't feel the need to hoard the extra as fat storage. You will, in effect, speed up your metabolism. This means that, even in a resting state, your body will start to burn more calories (use more fuel energy) in a day for normal function. The result is weight loss. For the rest of the biology behind the weight loss, we will next discuss exercise.

SHOULD YOU EXERCISE?

The first thing I want to cover here concerns male vs. female weight loss. If you are reading this, whether you are male or female, and you are on your own, this probably won't make any difference to you. But if you are female, and you are reading this with plans of making this change for both yourself and a male partner, I must warn you: a simple biological fact — that is not at all fair to us women — is that men store body fat and burn calories differently, and at a greater rate than we do. Men generally have more muscle mass, and they have the benefit of testosterone. Women tend to have less muscle mass than men, and by nature, our bodies are geared toward child-bearing; this means we already have a predisposed tendency to store more fat (to be later used as a source of extra energy for our pregnant bodies). Once you start this plan, you will see — whether you choose to exercise or not — that your male partner will tend to lose more weight than you, at a greater rate than you, especially in the first few months. All I can say is stick to the plan; you will eventually reach your goals. And now for some arguments in favor of exercise:

First, exercise means 'activity', and activity burns calories (energy / fuel). As I stated before, you must expend calories to lose weight. If you take in more calories than you expend, you will gain weight. If you eat roughly the same amount of calories as you expend in a day's time, you will maintain your current weight. The two ways to lose weight are to either eat fewer calories than you expend (in a resting state) in a days time, or to actively use more calories than you take in.

While just eating fewer calories will give you some resulting weight loss, there are things that you need to know. Once you start to lose a few pounds, especially when eating the right kinds of foods to make your body work more efficiently, you will start to have more energy. Why not put this new-found energy to good use, to help advance your weight loss? You don't have to take up an aerobics class or run a marathon. It can be an early morning or evening walk, especially to start.

Second, after you have lost between 10 and 20 pounds, you are going to notice some sagging. Your belly will sag; your love-handles will hang; if you are a woman, your breasts will most usually get smaller, and will have a tendency to sag as well. Light to moderate exercise in the beginning will not only burn more calories, helping your weight loss, but will help to tone and tighten your body along the journey.

Third, another advantage of exercise is the building and strengthening of muscle tissue. Muscle tissue burns more calories, even at rest. When you exert your muscles and give them exercise, making them stronger – and in some cases, should you choose, making them bigger – they become 'fat burning machines' within your body that will help you shed even more fat. Notice that I didn't say 'shed more pounds'. You may have heard this before, and it is true – muscle weighs more than fat. If you start building muscle, you may or may not lose weight, but you will lose fat and your body shape will change. The more muscle mass you have, the more calories your body will burn in a resting state.

Should you choose to include an exercise regimen in your weight-loss plan, only *you* can decide what works best for you. When I first started out, I had low energy, I had poor stamina, and because of years as a smoker, exertion caused difficulty in breathing. I knew I would have to start slow. I started with a Richard Simmons' *"Sweating to the Oldies"*® DVD. This was a very low-key, low impact, 30-minute aerobic workout. But the first time I tried it, I really did break a sweat, and thought I would barely make it through the entire video! I exercised to the video three times per week. After about a month, I realized that I was breezing through the video without the heavy breathing, without stopping for a water break, and without even breaking a sweat. At that time, I decided it was time to find something more challenging. I knew that my body needed exertion – something that would *raise my heart rate* – in order to burn calories and fat. I tried a gamut of different programs – some I purchased from the local store, others I ordered on-line. They ranged from low- to moderate-impact, to the outrageously insane. I tried Jillian Michaels videos, Zumba® dance, The Firm®, Weight Watchers® workout, The X-Factor®, and several from the Beach Body® video family, including Insanity®, Power 90®, Turbo Jam®, and Hip Hop Abs®.

For me, there was no comparison once I tried Turbo Jam® from Beach Body®. And *again*, I will *stress* to you here that I am *in no way* endorsing this as the program you should use, or encouraging or trying to entice you to purchase this program; I am simply stating that *this* was what I liked best; I felt like it was working for me and I could see results; and therefore, I stuck with it. You, as a consumer, need to do the same. You can watch sample videos of almost any workout program out there, on-line, before you buy them. You can get low-cost workout videos for around ten to 15 dollars from the sporting goods section of stores like WalMart or Target. If you prefer, you can join a local gym or aerobics center, and take step classes or HIIT (high intensity interval training) classes. You don't even have to do *any* of these programs. You can do simple calisthenics just as you learned all the way back in grade school – jump rope, jumping jacks, push-ups, sit-ups, running in place. You can use resistance bands / tubes, or free weights. Ride a bicycle. Play tennis with a friend. Jog around the block a few times, even. But in order to keep with it, you have to find what *you* like, and what you feel works best for *you*.

When I first approached my husband with my plan, and he agreed, I indicated to him my intent to exercise. He told me, in no uncertain terms, would he agree to exercise. He said I could change his diet however I wanted, but after working all day, he was tired, and his plan would be to come home and relax. I respected his decision and told him that was his choice. After the first month of changing only his diet, and after losing 20 pounds (yes, I said he lost 20 pounds in one month, *just* by changing his diet), he noticed what I said you probably will – everything was starting to sag. At that point, he decided he had better do something to start firming things up, as he still had quite a way to go in his weight-loss quest. Now, he is more regimented with his work-out program than I ever was. But we are both in better shape now than we were when we met almost 15 years ago.

As a final note to this chapter, I will say it once more: only *you* can decide if you will exercise, and what type of activity it will be. Whatever your decision, you have to be happy with the outcome or you will not stick with it.

WHAT DOES YOUR BODY NEED?

Up until this point, assuming you are overweight, you have been taking in more calories than you actually need to maintain your body weight. When you start taking in fewer calories – even when the goal is to lose – you may have a tendency, even when eating the six meals per day, to still feel hungry. So how do you find the right balance, or decide how many calories you need to consume each day, in order to start your weight loss journey?

In order to lose just one pound per week, you need a *daily deficit* of 500 calories. This means you either need to eat 500 calories less than your resting body needs per day to maintain your current body weight – OR – you need to *burn* 500 extra calories per day (through activity and exercise). To figure out how many calories you should eat in a day, consider the following formula:

1) Add a zero to the end of your current body weight; for instance, if you weight 200 pounds, you will start with 2000;

2) If you plan on starting an exercise regimen, add 20% for extra daily activity = 400; in this instance, you will start with 2400.

3) Subtract the 500 calorie deficit needed to lose one pound per week = 1900 calories per day.

4) If you are *not* planning on exercising, you will subtract the 500 calorie deficit needed from the original 2000 = 1500 starting calories per day.

Keep in mind that this formula does not take into account your body type or prior fitness level. If you already have some muscle tone, and are somewhat active, you may need to adjust your caloric intake slightly. The more overweight you are, as well as for being more sedentary, you may want to start with a slightly larger deficit. Once you start losing and become more active, you can add calories back in to fuel muscle gains.

I *very highly* recommend that in the beginning, you download some type of calorie counter app for your phone. I say this for the plain and simple reason that, as people, we have a tendency to lie to ourselves. We tell ourselves that "just one cookie" or "one small piece of candy" won't hurt, and we don't include those calories into our daily count. We tend to overestimate the calories we have burned, and underestimate the amount of calories we have consumed. In effect, we sabotage ourselves in our own diet plan.

Many available apps will not only calculate what you eat, but also what you burn in daily activity. At the same time, you still have to be *honest* with your entries into the app. By faithfully using the app, with every meal and every snack, you can see at a glance why you are – or are *not* – meeting your weight loss goals; and you can adjust your daily caloric intake accordingly.

Another bonus of using an app is that any time you make an entry, it will break each food item down for you. At the end of the day, you can tell in a glance what percentage of proteins, carbs, and fats you are consuming.

A good balance for weight loss and fat loss is a diet that consists of 35-40% protein, 30-40% carbohydrate, and around 20-25% (never more than 30%) fat.

Another easy way to combat hunger is to draw on one of your body's most basic and simple needs – *water*. For any weight-loss program, water is your best friend. Drinking water throughout the day will maintain hydration, fill you up and help stave off cravings, help prevent muscle cramps after exercise, and help flush the body of waste and toxins. You want to drink between 72-80 ounces of water per day.

You may want to consider taking supplements to start out, especially until you know that you are getting exactly what your body needs from your foods alone on a daily basis, to maintain a healthy balance. A good, overall multi-vitamin can ensure that your body will get all the vitamins and minerals it needs to function properly. Because most multi-vitamins contain much higher values of each vitamin and mineral than the body actually needs in a day's time, the best way to take a multi-vitamin is to get scored tablets and break them in half; take half in the morning, and half in the early evening. In this way, you get a higher benefit from the vitamin tablet, and your body doesn't flush all the excess vitamins / minerals away early in the day.

I also recommend getting a thorough check-up from your physician, and ask him or her to run a complete lab panel, as a baseline. You might already have some health problems that you are being monitored for, or that you might already be taking medication to treat. Do you know if you have any issues with your thyroid? Do you have high blood pressure or high cholesterol? Are you diabetic? These are things that you will want to consider when planning out menus for your diet plan, as well as deciding if you want to take any supplements.

When first starting out, I had lab work done, which indicated that my cholesterol was high. I had *never* had this issue before, and didn't think that I even had any health problems! I decided to also take a Fish Oil Supplement every day as well, along with my multi-vitamin. I went back to my doctor six months after changing my diet, and asked her to run my cholesterol again. My results were *amazing*! I had lowered both my "bad" and total cholesterol levels back to almost normal, in a mere six months, simply by changing the way I ate and taking one Fish Oil capsule per day!

You will want to take "progress" pictures and measurements before you start. You should dress in minimal clothing (boxers or shorts for males; bra and shorts, or bathing suit for females). Stand in front of a neutral background (such as a solid color wall), and take pictures of yourself – or have someone take them for you – facing forward, and also from the side. You want these to be full- or at least three-quarter-length pictures.

Wearing the same minimal clothing (or nothing at all), weigh yourself on an accurate bathroom scale. You can take a 10- or 15-pound weight and place it on the scale to check for accuracy. Write down the date and time of day that you measured your weight. You will want to *always* weigh yourself at the same time of day, every time you weigh. And always wear the same clothing (or nothing at all, if that is how you first weighed).

Using a standard cloth measuring tape, you will want to take and record the following measurements: chest; waist; hips; right and left mid-thigh; right and left upper arm (measure upper arm at the peak of the bicep). If you are male, you might also wish to measure your neck. Male or female, you might also want to measure the girth of your belly. These two measurements are optional, but for some (especially us women!), this belly measurement is as important as measuring the waist. I have included a weight and measurement grid where you can record your measurements, on page 66.

Once you change your eating habits, it is recommended that you do not weigh yourself more than once per week. Wearing the same clothes as before, take new pictures and measurements of yourself once per month. After you compare new results to those of the previous month, you can decide how to adjust your calorie intake to where you need to be to reach your goals.

THE SIMPLE PLAN

Here is the plain and simple plan that will start you on your road to healthy weight loss. For the first 30 days, be *strict* with yourself in following these simple rules:

NO eating out – period.

NO fried foods – period.

NO sodas – period.

NO processed meats, canned vegetables or fruits, or 'ready-made' meals (like frozen lasagna, frozen pizza, hamburger helper, canned soup, etc.).

Eat six meals per day – don't skip meals.

Eat healthy, fresh, balanced meals and snacks that are properly portioned.

NO snacking / 'cheating' between meals – not even *one* small piece of candy.

If you can do these seven things FOR 30 DAYS, you will start to see great changes in your body, and in your health. In the following pages, I am going to tell you what kinds of foods to eat and how to include them in your meal plan. The foods that will be included are going to help maximize your weight loss, and benefit your overall bodily functions (aiding with digestion and elimination, and helping to rid your body of toxins).

Focus on the "six-meals-per-day" aspect of the plan. Start by evaluating your lifestyle and work schedule. For example, my husband works during the day, while I work in the evenings. For us, we both eat on a relatively similar schedule:

7-8 AM	Breakfast
10 AM	Snack
Noon	Lunch
3 PM	Snack
5-6 PM	Dinner
8-8:30 PM	Snack

We try to never eat anything after 8:30 PM (or within two to three hours of going to bed). If you work at night, and sleep during the day, you will need to look at the hours you sleep / wake and adjust your "meals" accordingly for your waking times.

Limit carbs and fats as a "last meal" (snack). High protein snacks or shakes are the best options before sleep, as your body will process and break these down better in a resting state. Carbs and fats before bedtime tend to get stored.

Based on the schedule above, as well as figuring your caloric intake (see the chapter "What Does Your Body Need?"), based on a 1500-1900 calorie diet, you would want to distribute your intake over those six meals as follows:

Breakfast	300-350 calories
Morning snack	100-250 calories
Lunch	450-500 calories

Afternoon snack	150-250 calories
Dinner	300-350 calories
Evening snack	150-200 calories

You want to eat the major portion of your calories earlier in the day, so that you are using the energy you are feeding your body, through work and play and exercise, and not loading up on calories before bedtime, causing your body to 'store' that energy while you sleep.

Remember that the above is just an example. You will need to use the previously provided formula, to figure out your daily caloric need, based on your starting body weight and the amount of energy (exercise or routine daily activity) that you will expend while following this plan. You will then need to adjust your six-meals plan accordingly, by dividing your total allowance of calories over the day.

Stick to the plan and *do not cheat* for the first 30 days. After the first month, you can 'reward' yourself with a meal of your choice (home cooked or eating out). I think you will be very surprised at how you feel after eating that first "free meal"—we chose hamburgers and fries from a local drive-thru, and felt as if we had bricks in our stomachs after eating them!

Once you have survived your first 30 days of eating on the plan, and having your "free" meal, go right back to eating healthy. Allow yourself a "free" meal once every week or so; but make smarter choices when eating out—opt for soft tacos instead of hard-shell (fried tortilla) tacos; choose baked potatoes over fries. Limit (or skip) the breads served at many restaurants. And by all means, order smaller portions, or leave something on your plate! Maintain your calorie counts day by day, and watch the pounds start to come off.

One thing we need to discuss is a weight-loss

"plateau". A plateau happens when you are maintaining your calorie intake, and maybe you are or are not exercising, but your weight-loss seems to have stalled. You are well past your 30-day mark, but now you've been stuck at the same weight for a week or two without seeing any results. Something needs to change. At this point, you need to "jump start" your metabolism again.

One way to do this is to totally change the way you eat for a day. You've been following your plan, right? Okay. Have yourself a big, juicy steak and a baked potato with all the fixins, salad, buttery roll, maybe even a cold beer for dinner one evening. Or grab that deep-dish pepperoni pizza you've been wanting—have two or three slices. Then go right back into your plan the next day. Sometimes this throws a little kink in the armor, causing your body to say "hey, what was that?" Don't fret about it. It happens to all of us. Just don't use this "jump start" until you've finished the first 30 days of your plan.

In the next section, I will help you decide on what foods to choose for your plan, as well as tips on how to prepare them.

WHAT SHOULD YOU EAT?

As stated before, you want to eat a balanced diet. But how do you go about it? Eat whole grains, lean meats, and fresh fruits and vegetables. Make substitutions in your diet where you can for sugars and fats. Learn to *read labels*. Everything that says "low calorie" or "low fat" is not always the best choice!

You want to learn how to prepare your foods as well. Other than fresh, your best options are baked, steamed, or grilled. Remember—nothing fried in the first 30 days! For most of our meals, I use a double-decker "rice and vegetable" steamer. I use the bottom tray for meats (chicken, pork, or fish), and fill the top tray with fresh vegetable blends (such as diced zucchini, squash, and carrots; or a broccoli / cauliflower mix). You can get a good quality steamer for around $40 in department stores or online. Oster® has one that comes with two steaming trays, as well as a rice tray; but there are many others out there that will do the job.

Stock up on different types of seasonings, and limit (or skip) the salt! There are so many great seasoning combinations out there these days, you can make flavorful dishes without eating fried, greasy foods!

You want to choose lean cuts of pork, skinless chicken or turkey, fish filets, and ground turkey (in place of beef), or very lean cuts of beef in limited quantities (no more than two servings of beef per week).

Fill your diet with a variety of fresh, steamed, and grilled vegetables. You want to go heavy on green vegetables, such as broccoli, cabbage, Brussels sprouts, asparagus, sugar snap peas, snow peas, zucchini, spinach, and green beans. Baked yams make a great substitute for baked potatoes. Limit regular (white) potatoes to no more than once or twice per week. Steamed cauliflower can be grated as a substitute for "macaroni" and cheese; it can also be made into "hash browns"; mashed turnips can also substitute for mashed potatoes. Steamed carrots, squash, purple cabbage, yams (sweet potato), and corn can add some color and variety to your meals. Eat large salads alone, or add some grilled chicken and top with salsa or avocado.

Long-grain and wild or brown rice, quinoa, and semolina make great additions to any meal, as do most any beans. These grains, along with black beans, pinto beans, kidney beans, and navy beans, as well as split peas and lentils are packed with fiber and protein. Raw or roasted nuts, such as almonds, walnuts, peanuts, and cashews add protein and healthy fats; just beware of eating the 'flavored' and 'salted' kind—these add unwanted sugars and salt— stick with natural versions and you will be fine!

Limit pastas and white breads. Eat whole-grain breads (Sara Lee® makes a 45-calorie whole grain bread that has a wonderful taste and texture), or substitute wraps for sandwiches. You can also use large, fresh, lettuce leafs as a wrap and skip the bread altogether! Spaghetti squash can be used in place of traditional pasta noodles for spaghetti.

Almost any fresh fruit makes a great snack, but limit

fruit such as bananas—they can cause constipation and bloating. Berries (blueberries, strawberries, blackberries) make a great addition to breakfast cereals, oatmeal, and smoothies. Fresh peaches, apples, plums, oranges, pears, and melon can be eaten any time. Fresh grapefruit is a fat-burning friend! But beware—I'm not talking about the "old-fashioned" way of eating one, by slicing it in half, and slathering it with sugar! Peel and eat it like an orange—if you remove the thin 'skin' from each section, it greatly reduces the bitter taste associated with eating this helper fruit.

There are a multitude of other healthy choices out there for snacks as well. All natural peanut butter is a great choice; it is a healthy fat, is low in sodium, and is very filling. It also provides a great source of protein. The same goes for almond butter, or any of your nut butters, as long as you go with the 'natural' version. Greek yogurt cups and cottage cheese, with some added fresh berries make great snack foods or even breakfast items. You can also substitute Greek yogurt cream cheese as a spread for breakfast toast or English muffins—it has half the fat of regular cream cheese, but the taste is the same. Boiled eggs also make a great snack food high in protein. Veggie crisps (or chips) in place of potato chips will stave off those 'salty food' cravings. There are a variety of "popped" rice chips, as well as rice cakes that can be eaten plain or with a dab of peanut butter. Dried fruits (dehydrated apples, mango, bananas, raisins, etc.) make great snack foods.

Some fats are essential to a healthy diet, but you want to know which ones to eat. Olive oil is a great choice for cooking (I use olive oil cooking spray), or mixed with vinegar and spices for a salad dressing option. Avocado is a great, healthy fat to eat. You can mash ripe avocado with a dollop of olive-oil mayo and some seasonings to make a healthy spread for sandwiches, or to top off a salad. Substitute olive oil mayo for regular (or even low-fat) mayo; if you compare it to low-fat mayo, it is a better option because of the sugar content; and as a bonus, it *tastes* like regular mayo! As stated above, nuts not only provide a source of protein, but healthy fats as well. Fish (especially white fish) provide heart-healthy fats and essential oils. You also want some dairy fat, so opt for reduced or fat-free cheeses, but drink whole milk or 2%—not skim or fat-free milk.

Always remember, you want mainly a diet that consists of 35-40% protein, 30-40% carbohydrate, and around 20-25% (never more than 30%) fat.

SAMPLE MEALS AND MENUS

Here are some great sample meals / menus that show just how varied and tasty your diet can be, while still being healthy:

Day 1:			Approx. Calories
Breakfast	-	1/2 cup (dry) Plain oatmeal with 1/4 cup blueberries	
		Boiled egg	305
Snack	-	1 medium apple with	
		2 Tbs. all-natural peanut butter	265
Lunch	-	Steamed, seasoned chicken breast (4 oz) Steamed broccoli, cauliflower, & carrots	
		(2 cups)	270
Snack	-	Greek yogurt cup	110
Dinner	-	2 cups salad mix with chopped boiled egg Steamed or grilled salmon (4 oz) – chopped	
		1 Tbsp fat-free Ranch dressing	360
Snack	-	1 bag 100-calorie, single-serving	
		microwave popcorn	100

1410 Total

For the 1900 cal / day plan, you can increase your

breakfast oatmeal to 1 cup, increase chicken at lunch and salmon with dinner to 6 ounces, and add nuts with the yogurt snack mid-day. This will increase the total approximate calorie count to 1860. Make similar adjustments to other sample plans to get the daily calorie counts for your specific plan.

Day 2:			Approx. Calories
Breakfast	-	3/4 cup Special K cereal with	
		1/2 cup whole milk	170
Snack	-	Greek yogurt cup with added	
		fruit (in container)	125
Lunch	-	Steamed, seasoned pork loin chop (4 oz)	
		1 cup steamed Brussels sprouts	
		1/2 cup (cooked) brown rice	360
Snack	-	1/2 cup low fat cottage cheese	
		with 1/2 cup fresh strawberries	140
Dinner	-	Seasoned, grilled chicken breast (4 oz)	
		1 Medium baked yam with	
		1 Tbsp butter & cinnamon	
		1 ear corn on the cob	500
Snack	-	2 Tbsp all-natural peanut butter	
		with 5 Ritz crackers	270

1565 Total

Day 3:			Approx. Calories
Breakfast	-	2-egg omelet (made in non-stick	
		pan with olive oil cooking spray)	
		--use sliced mushrooms, low-fat grated	
		cheese, and chopped baby spinach	210
Snack	-	1 Quaker lightly salted rice cake with	
		2 Tbsp all-natural peanut butter	225
Lunch	-	Seasoned, grilled turkey burger patty with	
		fresh lettuce, tomato, onion	
		1 slice reduced-fat pepper jack cheese	

		Oro-wheat sandwich thin (round)	
		1 Tbsp spicy brown mustard	360
Snack	–	1 large grapefruit	100
Dinner	–	Baked spaghetti squash (1/4 squash) with 1 cup spaghetti sauce, cooked with turkey meatballs (from frozen) –	
		5 meatballs	345
Snack	–	1 bag 100-calorie, single-serving microwave popcorn	100

1340 Total

As you can see, varying your diet / menu choices will get you close to your day's calorie counts. There will be days when you will be just under, and other days where you will go just over your allotted calories. But if you stay right in that range, you will do just fine.

WATER, WATER, EVERYWHERE!

Okay, we've talked about what to eat, but what about what to drink? As I previously stated, when on any diet plan, water is your best friend. You still want to drink 72-80 ounces of water per day. Okay, I get it. You don't want to drink "just water" all the time. So what else can you have?

Your best choice, by far, is green tea. And I am not talking about the pre-bottled, sweetened (or even "diet" version of) green tea that you buy at the store. I am talking about pure, home-brewed (from a tea bag) green tea—plain and simple, or with a splash of lemon juice. There are several ways to go about this; one of which is to brew the tea bag(s) and add to a pitcher of water, or use the single-serving bags in a bottle of water. It isn't really necessary to "brew" the green tea. I like the flavored green tea bags from Lipton® with Açai fruit; I frequently pop one of these into a bottle of water, put the lid back on and pop it into my lunch bag. After an hour or two in the fridge at work, it's ready for me to drink. I just pull the tea bag out and throw it in the trash, and drink my tea. I will often add a splash of lemon juice to the water before adding the tea bag. I still drink my water, though, as even though green tea is good for you, it is also a diuretic, and you don't want to get dehydrated. Drink it three or four times a week, and don't make it your first choice over water.

Another good choice (and we go back to the great, "fat-burning" properties of grapefruit) is grapefruit juice. You can choose pink or white, or reduced-calorie (we drink the Ocean Spray® Light-50, which is 50 calories per serving); just don't drink more than one serving per day of this as well.

Stay away from other fruit juices in general. Unless you fresh-squeeze them yourself, they tend to be loaded with sugar, and you are just adding "empty calories" back into your diet. Remember to add in any drink calories into your calorie-tracker app as well; even though they are not 'food', they still count!

Limit coffee intake to no more than 1-2 cups per day, and preferably in the morning. By drinking mainly water and green tea (which is naturally decaffeinated), you will sleep better by limiting your caffeine intake to first thing in the morning. If you don't drink black coffee, look at what you are putting into your coffee each morning. Do you use cream? What about sugar? Every single teaspoon of each of these *counts* toward your daily total. I didn't realize how many "empty calories" I was putting into my fat body every morning until I started to track it; three teaspoons of sugar (30 calories) and two teaspoons of powdered creamer (70 calories) made each cup of coffee a whopping 100 calories! I found a flavored, liquid creamer that tastes the same as what I was adding to my cup each morning, for a 35-calorie serving, so I cut each cup of coffee by two-thirds the calories. By limiting myself to two servings, I was able to cut my caloric intake (just with coffee alone!) by 130 calories a day!

While an occasional glass of wine or a mixed drink with dinner is just a-okay, you do want to stay away from alcohol in general. Beer is your biggest offender—the wheat and hops and barley just add on empty carb calories that you really don't need! There's a reason they call it a "beer belly".

Smoothies make a great drink as a meal or snack replacement. You can make these in a regular blender or a specialty blender (such as a Magic Bullet®, Nutri-Bullet®, or Ninja®). As long as you make these fresh as well (and don't use the frozen smoothie mixes, or pre-bottled smoothie drinks), you can reap the benefits of all the vitamins and minerals from the fresh fruits and vegetables you use. I have included a few of my favorite smoothie and drink recipes in the recipes section.

BESIDES WEIGHT LOSS, WHAT'S IN IT FOR ME?

Of course, you are reading this book because your main goal is to lose weight, right? But did you know that there are many other benefits of following this healthy eating plan?

Do you ever eat a meal at lunchtime, then return to work and get the "bobble-head", trying to stay awake mid-afternoon? This is because most people tend to skip breakfast, and then eat a high fat, high carbohydrate lunch, which causes a severe spike in blood sugar. After it peaks, your blood sugar will plummet, leaving you feeling tired and run-down. When your blood sugar drops, you will more likely experience cravings, and by mid-afternoon you'll be looking for something sweet—a candy bar or a piece of left-over cake from the office birthday party. This drives your blood sugar up once again, starting the cycle all over. Eating six, properly-proportioned meals (traditional meals plus snacks) throughout the day, helps to maintain a steady blood glucose level in your body. This means you will be less prone to experience those "highs" and "lows" that most people are so familiar with. This also means less cravings, and over-eating (by snacking) as a result.

Have you ever heard those commercials on TV that

announce "most people are carrying around between 15-20 pounds of excess waste in their colon?" They advertise a "miracle pill" that helps your body get rid of this excess waste. Well, guess what? Eating fresh fruits and vegetables—especially green, leafy vegetables, such as spinach, kale, asparagus, and broccoli—will add fiber to your diet and help move all of that stuff along your digestive tract. If you follow this plan, you *will* notice a change in your bowel habits; and you *will* be getting rid of that excess waste they are talking about in those commercials. If you have trouble with bloating and constipation already, you will want to take it easy, at the start, with the green vegetables (especially broccoli and cabbage), because they can make you 'gassy'. But increase them each day in your diet until you are eating full servings, and they will rid you of that constipation problem very quickly. In the recipe section, I have included recipes for a "spinach smoothie" and a "detox tea" that will both help speed things up in that department.

Do you have high blood pressure? Diabetes? High cholesterol? The benefits of this plan are multiple. Weight loss will naturally help with all of these. As I stated previously, the benefits of eating six meals throughout the day will help maintain your blood sugar level at a more steady state throughout the day. Eating the right fats (healthy fats, from olive oil, fish, and nuts) will help lower your cholesterol levels, as well as your blood pressure. Using alternative seasonings and trimming back on salt will help with your blood pressure as well.

Above all else, as you start to eat as outlined in this plan, you will not only look better, you will feel better! Getting the right vitamins and minerals into your body, maintaining a steady blood sugar level, and not eating greasy, fried foods, along with ridding your body of built-up toxic wastes will leave you with more energy and drive! You will also feel better because you will sleep better, and awaken feeling rested and refreshed each day.

THE "NATURAL" CHOICE

Some may disagree with me, but my thoughts about substitutions are this: anything that is natural is healthier for you than the imitation.

Therefore, I prefer to use natural sugar over artificial sweeteners (the only exception to this is if you are diabetic, and your physician has instructed you to NOT use real sugar). Otherwise, *limit* the amount of sugar that you use, but use real sugar.

Butter is better than margarine (if you don't believe me, put a tub of butter and a tub of margarine out on the counter and let them sit there until they are no longer solid; then put them back into the fridge and see what happens!).

I like real mayo, but it is high in fat. Low-fat mayo is high in sugar, and doesn't taste the same. Olive oil mayo has better fat, no extra sugar, and tastes like 'real' mayo.

Fresh fruits and vegetables are always the best option. After that, go with frozen—but only with natural fruits and veggies—don't get the frozen vegetable "dinners" that are swimming in butter or "sauce". Canned is a last resort—canned / jarred fruits are often packed in syrup and loaded with sugar and calories. Canned / jarred fruits and vegetables contain higher salt, sugar, and preservative content than frozen.

Use fresh or frozen meats that are in their "pure" form; this means chicken, turkey, fish, and cuts of pork or beef that are not cured, smoked, processed, or canned. Avoid luncheon meats like the plague! And, yes—I'm going to say it—this means avoiding bacon as well! Bacon and sausage should be eaten no more than once a week, and not until you've passed your first 30 days on the plan! Whenever possible, avoid canned or processed meats. I eat canned tuna sparingly and only packed in water—never tuna packed in oil!

Eat those foods that you can without adding anything to them. Buy healthy cereals and eat them without adding sugar. Add fresh or dried fruit to cereal or oatmeal—but beware that some dried fruits have added sugar as well—read the labels!

There has been a big push lately toward "gluten free" products. Unless you have celiac disease, or gluten intolerance, if you limit your white flour intake you shouldn't have a problem. Stick with whole-grain breads and pastas, and eat portion-sizes only, keeping track of your calories. Use substitutions, such as cauliflower, eggplant, and spaghetti squash for pastas. You can find great substitution recipes on the internet, and I have included some in the recipes section of this book as well.

SOME FINAL THOUGHTS

Please remember that real change takes time. For any change to become a habit, you need to give it at minimum, 30 days. Follow this plan for 30 days, and you *will* start to see changes. But remember that everyone's body is different. Some of you will see small changes in the first 30 days, while others will see dramatic differences. For those of you that only see small changes in the beginning, don't lose hope, and don't give up! Small change is *still* change!

Like I said in the beginning, I cannot make you a promise to lose "x" amount of weight in "x" amount of days. This is merely a starting point. YOU have to make the decision to follow through. YOU have to make your own plan, based on this starting point, and carry out that plan.

Eat *clean*. Drink your *water*. Keep a food diary, or use an app to track your calories—treat it like a religion, and write down (or log) everything you put in your mouth! If you choose to exercise, find something you can *stick* with, and just do it! Track your progress—weigh yourself weekly, and take monthly measurements and pictures.

Be aware that plateaus will happen. Adjust your diet and get over that hump, to jump start your weight loss again.

Don't be afraid to try new things! If you've never eaten broccoli, don't say you don't like it without giving it a real try! You might like it better fresh, rather than steamed, or vice-versa, but give it a try first. This goes for any new foods you might introduce into your diet on this plan. Things that sound weird to the ear can have a much different take on the pallet! Eggplant... okra... squash... turnips... lentils... beets... spinach. There are so many good foods out there, if you keep an open mind and give them a try!

I know a lot of what I have said may seem repetitive, *but*—you must say this over and over to yourself. I *will* drink my water. I *will* eat clean. I *will* track my calories. I *will* watch my portions.

Your old mantra may have been "I can do this." Let your new mantra be "I *will* do this!"

The timing will vary for each person, but after the first 30 days, you will start to "get the hang of it." For some, it might take a while longer, but eventually, you will not have to weigh or measure or portion out your food. You can look at your plate and *know* when you have the right portions for a meal. You will be able to choose and grab healthy snacks without having to measure every bite. The discipline in the beginning will become your habits of the future.

I know I told you in the beginning that you don't have to give up your favorite foods to do this... and you don't. After your first 30 days on the plan, you can "reward" yourself once or twice a month with a dinner out. Just make the right choices. Eat *two* slices of a medium pizza, instead of devouring an entire large pie. When that waitress comes around at the Mexican food restaurant with that second basket of chips and salsa while you wait, say "no, thank you!" Leave food on your plate. Most restaurant meal portions are double, or even triple, what a normal serving size is! Order from the kid's menu. Eat at a buffet where you can make the right choices (more salads, greens, and other veggies). Order the grilled chicken instead of that which is breaded and fried.

I wish each and every one of you good luck on your journey. Here's hoping for as much success to you, as we have had in our own weight-loss journey.

BEFORE AND AFTER

Anyone that knows me and my husband personally, you have seen the changes first-hand, over the past two years. For those of you that don't know us, here is a glimpse of the changes we have gone through:

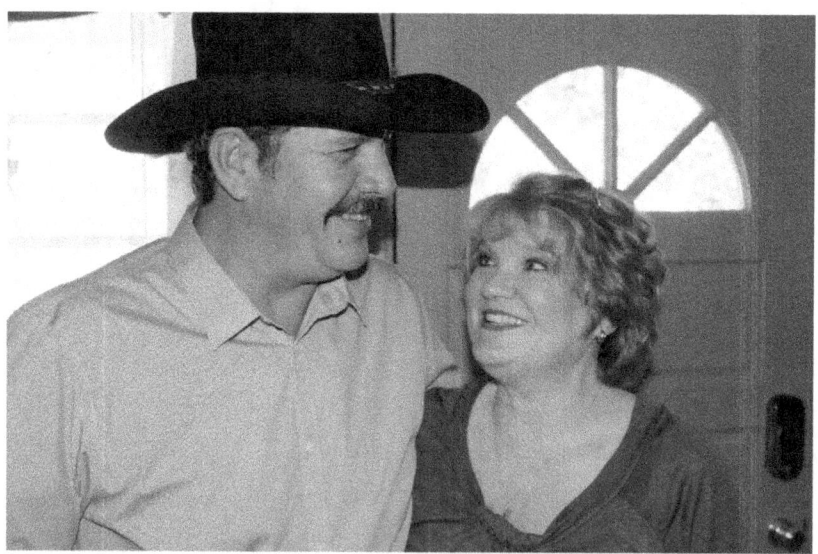

This is the picture that changed my life. We were going to my cousin's wedding, and after I saw this picture, I knew it was time to make a change.

This was in February of 2013. At my heaviest ever (without being pregnant), I was 180 pounds. My husband was pushing 260.

The following pictures were taken on my birthday, in December 2012; I was almost as heavy as in February (previous picture). One year later, I put on the same outfit to show my progress! The weight loss shows in my face as well!

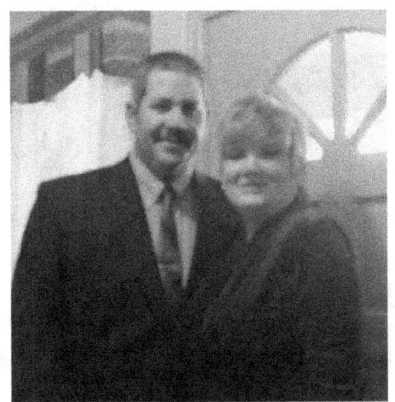
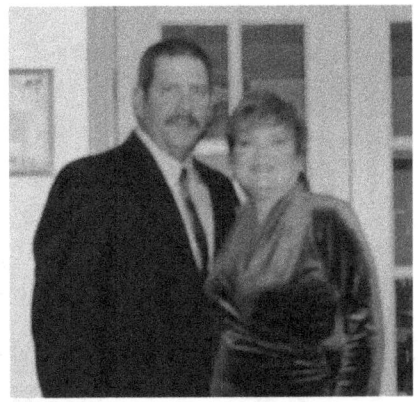

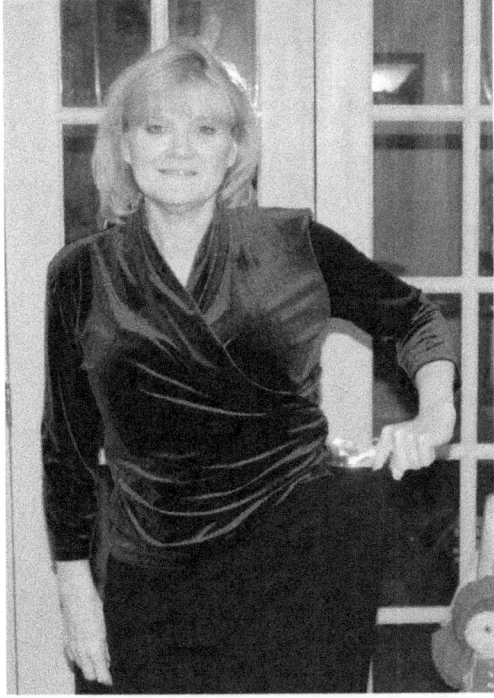

I was so proud to take this picture. I am holding the waistband of this skirt almost six inches from my waist! The blouse is also draped the way it should be, and not straining against my form!

The following pictures were taken at the Fire Department Christmas Dinner, in December of 2012, and again in December of 2013. Remember that we started this eating program in March of 2013, so our weight loss was over a period of nine months. My husband was so proud of his "before" and "after", that he couldn't wait to get to that dinner and take another picture with the same firefighter from his department as the previous year, as a comparison:

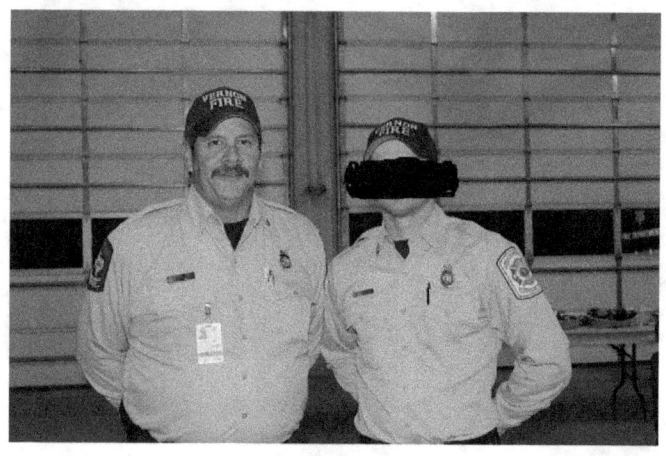

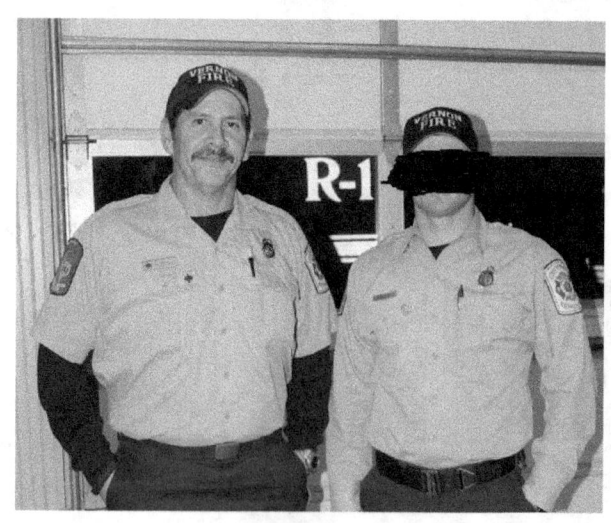

These next two pictures were taken in 2014; one at the Fire Department's Formal Banquet, and one was a photo shoot that my husband and I did, just to have some pictures of the new "us". And guess what? No crying / tears on shopping trips for these events!

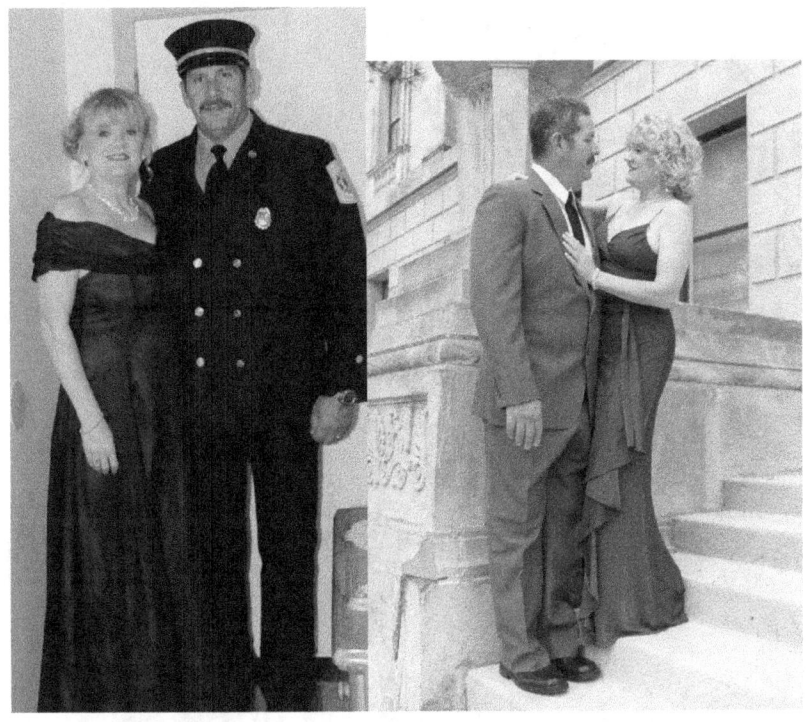

I think it important for me to note here, that while our bodies were going through these changes, we had to buy clothing several times. As anyone knows, this *can* get expensive!

For months, we shopped at Goodwill® and other second-hand stores for bargain clothing, so we would not break the bank on clothes, or walk around with our pants falling off of us.

It's a personal preference, but as you start losing the pounds, you will need some options, so keep that in mind.

These final pictures I'm going to show you are from my first book's photo shoot, in 2012, right before "The Envelope" was released, and again in 2014, before the release of "Burn." It's something to be excited over the release of your first novel, and having a publisher tell you they need photos for your book and for marketing purposes. But I *hated* the way I looked in those first photos!

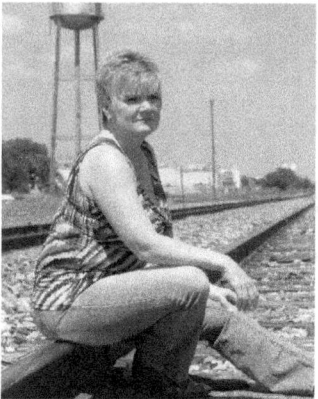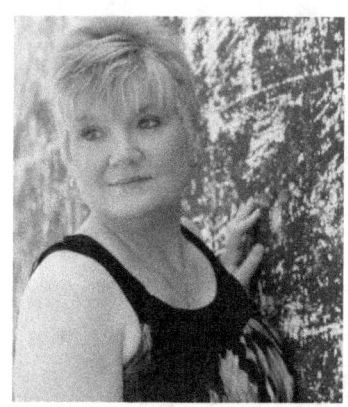

When I had the chance for a "do-over" with my second novel, I jumped at it, and I loved the way those pictures turned out:

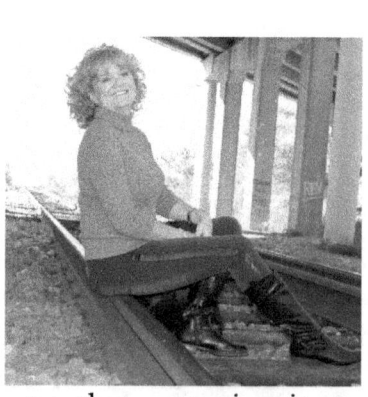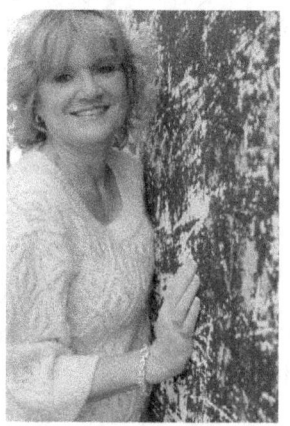

I hope that you give it your all, and follow the plan. And in the end, I hope you are as happy with your results as we are with ours! Now on to some recipes!

RECIPES

In these final pages, I am going to share with you some of the recipes I used in fixing healthy, delicious meals for our weight-loss journey.

Not only did I use these recipes on our way to losing the weight, but we still continue to eat them today.

A note here about seasonings: I may refer to a specific seasoning in a recipe, or I may just say "seasoned". I have an entire array of various seasonings in my kitchen cabinet, and I use different seasonings each time I make the same meal (or variation of).

Three things I will not do without are black pepper, garlic powder, and Butter Buds®. I also use olive oil cooking spray for almost everything!

Just keep in mind that you have to use seasonings that suit your taste... just limit your salt so you are not retaining water (and water weight!). Experiment with your own blend of seasonings and spices, and find the ones that you and your family enjoy the most.

Enjoy these recipes, and find some of your own. Open up your web browser and type "healthy recipes" in the search box. There are hundreds of recipe sites where you can find delicious, easy-to-prepare meals right at home.

Keeping some variety in your diet will ensure that you don't get "bored", or start having cravings that make you stray from your plan.

My Favorite Smoothie:

Ingredients:
   1 cup baby spinach leaves
   1 medium banana
   5 strawberries
   1 cup coconut water

Directions:
   Wash spinach leaves and place in blender; cut up the banana and wash / cut up strawberries, placing them on top of the spinach. Add coconut water, and blend on high speed until smooth. Drink cold.

Tips:
   I make these up ahead of time by taking a large bag of baby leaf spinach, washing & draining it, and putting 1-cup servings in freezer bags. I then add my chopped fruit, seal the bags and freeze. When I plan a smoothie into my day's meals, I take a bag out of the freezer and let it thaw (30-45 minutes, or in the refrigerator over night).
   You can also use different fruits for different flavor combinations. Mango, pineapple, berries, and melons make good smoothie ingredients. You can also buy frozen, chopped fruit pieces to use in these, which makes them quick and easy.

My Favorite Protein Smoothie:

Same as above, but after a workout, I add a scoop of whey isolate protein powder after the fruit, before the coconut water.

Steamed Chicken Breast:

Ingredients:
    Boneless, skinless chicken breasts (fresh or frozen)
    Olive oil cooking spray   Seasonings

Directions:
    Spray surface of chicken breasts lightly with olive oil cooking spray; sprinkle on desired seasonings and place in bottom tray of steamer. Steam cook for 35-45 minutes (takes longer for frozen).

Tips:
    Choose seasonings that go with the combination of vegetables you are using. For example, use Italian seasoning when serving with baby potatoes and sugar snap peas; use an Asian-style seasoning when serving with asparagus and rice.
    Use this same method of cooking for steamed, boneless pork loin chops, and fish fillets. Pork takes about 35 minutes in the steamer, while fish will only take 20-25 minutes from frozen.
    Adjust your cooking times to correspond with your vegetables. Vegetables do not take as long to steam as meats (except for fish), so when cooking chicken or pork, you will want to add your upper steam basket of vegetables when you have about 20-25 minutes left to go; you can generally add your vegetables at the same time you start fish, but times will vary depending upon the steamer you are using.
    I don't recommend using the steam method for beef; it has a higher fat content, which tends to muck up the steamer, and it curls and becomes tough. Beef is better when broiled, baked, or grilled.

Steamed Vegetables

Ingredients:
    2 cups (per serving) any vegetable combination
    Olive oil cooking spray   Butter Buds
    Seasonings

Directions:
    Place vegetables in upper steamer basket and rinse / drain. Spray lightly with olive oil cooking spray. Sprinkle with Butter Buds butter-flavored sprinkles, and desired seasonings. Place lid on basket, and shake lightly to blend seasonings. Place steamer basket on top of lower steam basket (steaming meats) when your meat has approximately 20-25 minutes left to cook.

Tips:
    Some grocery stores have pre-bagged, fresh vegetables in combination packages, such as broccoli/cauliflower mix, broccoli/cauliflower/carrot mix, snow peas/carrots mix, etc. These are very convenient, and keep you from having to buy each vegetable separately, then clean and chop before preparing.
    Some of our favorite steamed vegetable combinations are:
                Baby (nugget) potatoes with green beans
                    Sugar snap peas with carrots
                Broccoli, cauliflower, and carrots
    Asparagus spears with cubed yellow squash & zucchini

    If you have a grilling basket, the same method of preparation works great for vegetables, and place them on the grill instead of steaming, if you plan to cook out on the grill.

Spaghetti Squash with Sauce

Ingredients:
    1 large spaghetti squash   Italian seasoning
    Olive oil cooking spray   Garlic powder
    1 jar spaghetti sauce
    1 bag frozen turkey meatballs, or 1 lb roll ground turkey

Directions:
    Preheat oven to 350°.

    Using a sharp knife, cut the stem off the end of the squash; cut the squash in half. Scoop out the inside center (which looks much like a cantaloupe). Spray each half with olive oil cooking spray. Sprinkle with garlic powder and Italian seasoning. Place both halves cut-side *down* on a foil-lined baking sheet or shallow pan. Cover tightly with foil, and bake in oven for 35-40 minutes.

    While squash is baking, prepare your sauce. Place five meatballs (per person served) in a skillet (or brown the ground turkey and drain). Heat meatballs over medium-high heat until outsides start to brown. Add sauce of choice and turn heat down to medium. Cover and simmer until meatballs are heated thoroughly.

    Remove squash from oven. Using an oven mitt, carefully pick up one half of the squash. Holding it over a plate or serving bowl, use a fork to rake down the insides of the squash. The squash will "string out" onto the plate and have the appearance of spaghetti noodles. Cover with one cup sauce / 5 meatballs per person served.

Tips:
    One half of a spaghetti squash is considered a "serving". We have never been able to eat this much, so

one half feeds both of us for one meal. Scrape the other half out into a storage container for later use, as the squash will not "string" as well once it is cold.

Use whatever spaghetti sauce you prefer, but remember to read your labels! Many of them are much higher in sugar content that others. I prefer to use most any of the Bertolli® sauces, or Newman's Own®, as they have a lower sugar content.

Quick and Easy Alfredo Sauce

Ingredients:
  1 stick butter   2 cups fat-free Half-and-half
  1 – 8 oz package Greek yogurt cream cheese
  2 tsp garlic powder   1 Tbsp black pepper
  6 oz grated, reduced-fat Parmesan cheese

Directions:
  Melt butter and cream cheese in a saucepan over medium low heat, stirring frequently. Add garlic powder, and stir in cream, a little at a time, with a wire whisk, to get out any lumps. Stir in Parmesan and pepper; remove from heat when sauce reaches desired consistency. Sauce will thicken rapidly if cooked too long.

Tips:
  This is a low-fat version of a classic sauce, that tastes so delicious, no one will believe you when you tell them it is low fat! This can be served over the spaghetti squash as well; add a grilled or steamed chicken breast, chopped into pieces, to make a great Chicken Alfredo.

  You can serve this over traditional pasta noodles as well. Just remember to watch your carbs – opt for gluten-free noodles, or "vegetable" noodles when you can!

Italian Baked Chicken

Ingredients:
    Desired # of boneless, skinless chicken breasts
    Low-fat Mozzarella cheese slices
    Olive oil cooking spray   Garlic powder
    Italian seasoning
    1 small jar pizza sauce

Directions:
    Preheat oven to 350°.
    Place chicken breasts in a baking dish. Spray lightly with cooking spray. Season with Italian seasoning and garlic powder to taste. Bake 35-40 minutes, until almost done. Remove from oven and cover each breast with a slice of cheese. Pour pizza sauce over all breasts, and return to oven. Bake 5-7 more minutes, until cheese is melted and sauce begins to bubble.

Mashed Turnips

Ingredients:
    1 lb turnips, peeled and diced (large cubes)
    2-3 Tbsp butter   Salt   Pepper
    1 tsp sugar

Directions:
    Bring a large pot of salted water to a boil over high heat. Once boiling, add turnips and cook for 20-30 minutes until tender. Drain and return back to pot. Add butter, sugar, pepper, and salt. Mash with potato masher to desired consistency. Serve in place of mashed potatoes. (Adjust seasonings according to your taste; I found this to be too sweet, so next go-round, I omitted the sugar).

Spinach Lasagna

Ingredients:
  1 lb ground turkey   Fresh chopped spinach
  Minced garlic   Italian seasoning
  Shredded, reduced-fat Mozzarella cheese
  Reduced-fat Parmesan cheese
  Reduced-fat Ricotta cheese (small container)
  Sliced mushrooms (optional)
  Marinara sauce
  Lasagna noodles (I use the gluten free)

Directions:

Boil lasagna noodles until al dente. Remove from heat and rinse with cold water to avoid overcooking. Let drain.

Brown ground turkey with garlic and Italian seasoning in a pan. When done, add two-thirds of the marinara sauce.

Chop fresh spinach and mince 2-3 garlic cloves; put in a bowl & toss together.

Place a layer of noodles in the bottom of a casserole dish. Cover with half the meat mixture. Spoon on Ricotta cheese. Layer on spinach/garlic mixture (squeeze liquid out of the spinach with your hands first, or you will have soggy lasagna!). Add mushrooms here (if you are using them). Sprinkle with Mozzarella. Add another layer of noodles and repeat all layers.

Top with a final layer of noodles. Cover with remaining one-third of the sauce, and sprinkle the top with Parmesan.

Bake at 350° for about 20 minutes, until all the cheeses and sauce starts to bubble.

You can also make this minus the ground turkey for a vegetarian lasagna that is still just as good!

Shredded Chicken and Black Bean Tacos

Ingredients:
  4 boneless, skinless chicken breasts
  1 jar salsa (try to use all-natural)
  Seasonings (I use poultry seasoning, cumin, oregano,
      and garlic powder)

Directions:
  Slow-cook: Mix all ingredients together in a crock pot and cook until done.
  Fast-cook: Boil chicken breasts with seasonings until done; drain, chop, and mix with salsa.
  Serve in steamed corn tortillas with black beans and fresh guacamole or avocado spread.

Tips:
  You can use fresh cooked black beans, or canned. If you make fresh black beans, they take a *long* time to cook (longer than pinto beans and other beans). If you use canned black beans, open the can and dump the beans into a colander. Rinse with cold water to remove all the packing juice, which contains a lot of salt. Place the beans in a small sauce-pan and add one can of water back to the beans before heating.

Grilled Squash

Ingredients:
  Yellow and zucchini squash   Seasonings
  Olive oil cooking spray

Directions:
  Wash all squash thoroughly and cut ends off. Slice the

squash lengthwise, about one-quarter inch thick. Spray the slices lightly with olive oil cooking spray, and sprinkle with desired seasonings.

Place on hot grill, grilling about 7-10 minutes, until browned and tender.

Tips:

Use this method for grilling asparagus as well. Use whatever spices you desire to your taste preference.

"Dry" Fried Egg or Omelet

Use a small, non-stick fry pan and olive oil cooking spray to make "fried" eggs or fluffy omelets without using butter or oil.

You get the benefits of the proteins in eggs, without the added fats. They are just as delicious!

Detox Tea

Ingredients:
    Water   Lemon juice
    Yogi detox tea bag   Cranberry juice

Directions:

In an empty 20 oz water bottle or other container, mix 4 oz cranberry juice with a few drops of lemon juice. Fill with water, and add the tea bag. Let chill in refrigerator for 2-3 hours. Remove the tea bag and drink. This will rid your body of toxins and "help clean out the pipes".

§

I could continue to list countless, healthy recipes I have

found and used in the past two years. However, each and every one of you is going to have to make your own choices on this journey.

Research on the internet; look for "healthy recipes" and find those you can live with, within your food tastes and preferences.

Just remember to avoid anything fried, practice portion control, and don't starve yourself! Eat your six meals per day!

An Honest "Before" and "After" Record			
	Month 1	Month 2	Month 3
Weight			
Chest			
Waist			
Belly			
Hips			
Right Mid-Thigh			
Left Mid-Thigh			
Right Upper Arm			
Left Upper Arm			
	Month 4	Month 5	Month 6
Weight			
Chest			
Waist			
Belly			
Hips			
Right Mid-Thigh			
Left Mid-Thigh			
Right Upper Arm			
Left Upper Arm			

Use the table above to track your results. Be sure to record your measurements every month, and take your monthly progress pictures.

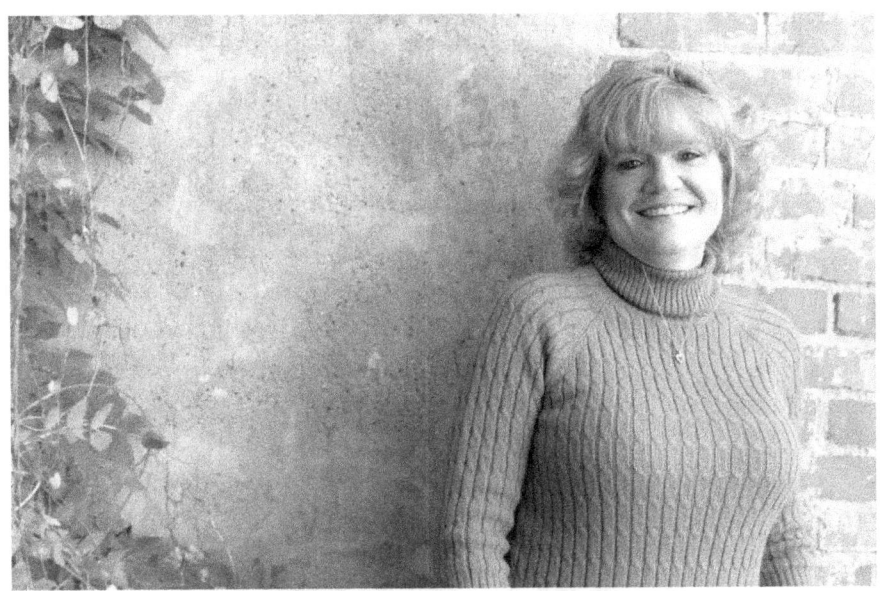

ABOUT THE AUTHOR

R. Sue Oleson was born and raised in Texas, at the gateway of Tornado Alley. A graduate of New Mexico State University, she is a Registered Nurse, and has worked in both acute & long-term care, rehab, and psychiatric nursing.

She enjoys watching movies and reading a good book--ANY good book! While crime and mystery novels are her favorites, she grew up sneaking her mom's romance novels—hence, her natural gravitation toward writing romantic suspense. She has three published fiction novels in the Romantic Suspense genre – "The Envelope", "Burn", and "Fatal Desire".

When not writing, she also enjoys singing Karaoke, relaxing in the pool, and taking motorcycle trips with her husband. Still living in Tornado Alley, she & her husband are both licensed Amateur (HAM) Radio Operators, and are active in local Emergency Management / Storm Spotting for the community.

This is the first non-fiction book by this author.

www.RSueOleson.net

Follow me on Facebook: https://www.facebook.com/RSueOleson
or Twitter: https://twitter.com/rsueoleson

***

CONTACT ME:
rsueoleson@gmail.com

OTHER WORKS FROM THIS AUTHOR

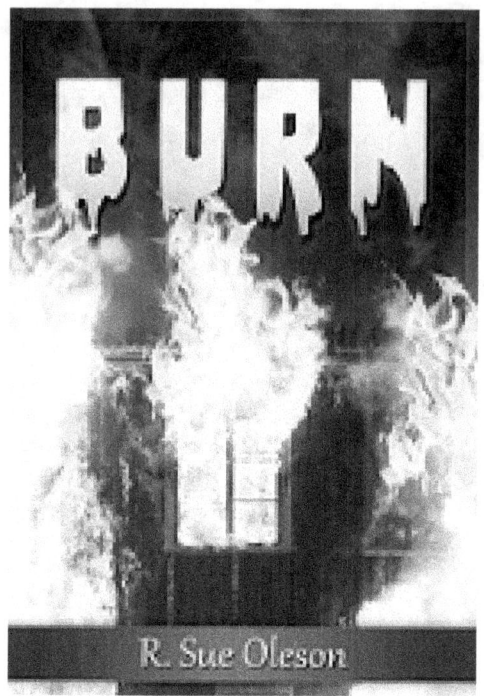

There's an arsonist in the city, and he means business. But Captain Nick Calhoun, a fourth-generation firefighter, can't seem to keep his mind on the game. He's too busy trying to drink away a bad memory. When his behavior puts his department—and his men—in jeopardy, the fire chief has no choice but to give him an ultimatum: work with a co-captain until he can regain control, or lose his job.

When Nick agrees, he is ready for anything but Danni O'Brien. Danni is a female firefighter, and the most beautiful woman Nick has ever laid eyes on. There's something about her that Nick is instantly drawn to, and he wants to get closer. But Danni is hiding a dark secret of her own; a secret that forces her to keep Nick—and all men—at bay.

As the sparks between them fly, a fire hits close to home, and they are forced to work against time to try and stop a madman. When tensions smolder, can Nick and Danni let go of their pasts long enough to stop the destruction? Or will they crash and burn in the fire of their own memories?

***** "...paints a vivid look into the life of arson investigation and firefighters."

**** "A fiery hot romantic thriller..."

***** "Hard to put down..."

OTHER WORKS FROM THIS AUTHOR

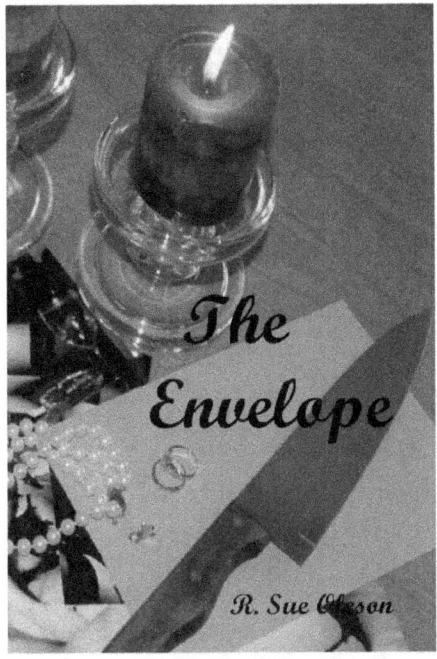

Carol Long has a life most people only dream of—a large estate in a gated community, designer clothes, a luxury sports car, and high-ranking status on society's ladder. But Carol isn't happy; in fact, she suspects her very handsome and very successful husband is cheating on her. Soon after she hires a private investigator to find proof of his indiscretions, Doug Long turns up dead, and Carol finds herself accused of his murder.

Enter Detective Ben Anderson—a strictly no-nonsense and by-the-book cop. When Ben crosses paths with the beautiful and wealthy Mrs. Long, he doubts her story from the start. But when they are thrust together in a turn of events, he soon finds himself lusting after his latest murder suspect, causing him to doubt his own instincts.

Just how far will Ben be willing to go in his quest for the truth? Will he cross the line of the law, risking his entire career—and maybe even his own life—to save her?

**** "A page-turner of a romantic suspense. From page one... I found it hard to put down."

***** "Amazing! ...Plot keeps you on your toes and guessing!"

***** "Riveting! ...Kept my attention to the end!"

OTHER WORKS FROM THIS AUTHOR

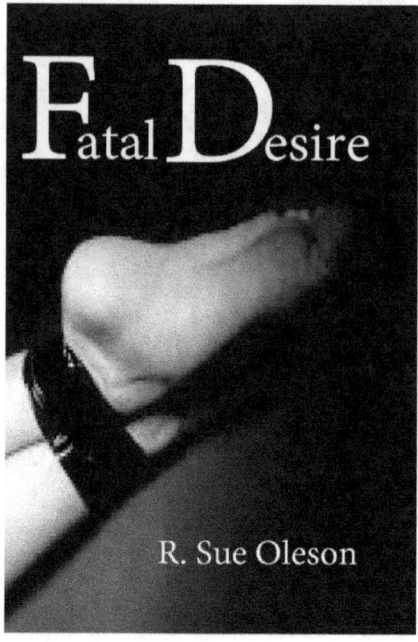

Stress is running high in the Rose Hill Police Department. There's a serial killer on the loose, and the clock is ticking away toward his next kill. The pressure is on to stop him, but with next to nothing to go on, Detective Stevie Monahan is just spinning her wheels.

But how can you track down a ghost of a killer, when you're dealing with ghosts of your own? All Stevie wants to do is catch this guy, but life keeps getting in the way—and so does her partner, Blake Bower. As Stevie watches her case unravel, she feels the need to unwind—landing her right in the clutches of handsome playboy bartender, Geoffrey Nichols.

But is Geoffrey hiding his own dark secrets? Blake seems to think so, but Stevie doesn't want to hear it. As the tension between them builds, can they continue to work together, and try to stop the madman wreaking havoc on their once-sleepy, suburban town, or will Blake drive Stevie right into the waiting arms of a killer?

**** "...sick, twisted, and original! Couldn't put it down!"

Released February 2015